Healing With Nature Workbook: for children, parents and others too

By Michael R. Basso

I0410055

~ 2 ~

About the Author

Michael has written and co-authored a variety of children's books designed to build tolerance, respect and wellness. Michael has written more than 150 popular articles on wellness and holistic health. Dr. Basso has also written for the Yale Journal for the Humanities in Medicine as well as professional articles in Psychiatry and Neuroscience.

Michael R. Basso has significant experience as a leader in quality and reliability engineering and management in industry, as well as being a college level educator in psychology at Yale University and the University of Connecticut. His experience also includes being a consultant, researcher, and newspaper columnist. Michael is the president of the Connecticut Holistic Health Association.

Dr. Basso has a Ph.D. in professional psychology and biomedical systems, an MS in engineering science, and an MBA with a focus in executive leadership and an interdisciplinary Professional Development Diploma in pathophysiology, neural systems, and education. He also holds a BS in electrical engineering. Michael is certified in quality and reliability engineering and quality auditing, as well as variety of health related areas

~ 3 ~

What a glorious day!

The day was wonderful. Belle had climbed a mountain, swam across the lake and even ate the best vegetarian meal ever – all things that were important to her this year.

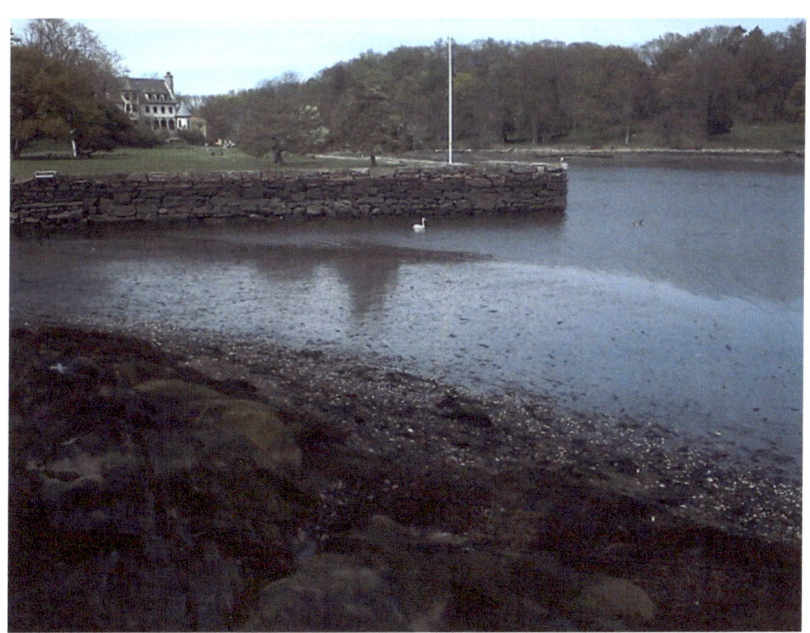

As she climbed into her sleeping bag, she decided to pray to God to teach her the 'coolest' things on her vacation.

Just then in her dream, she saw a beautiful gull with a special feather.

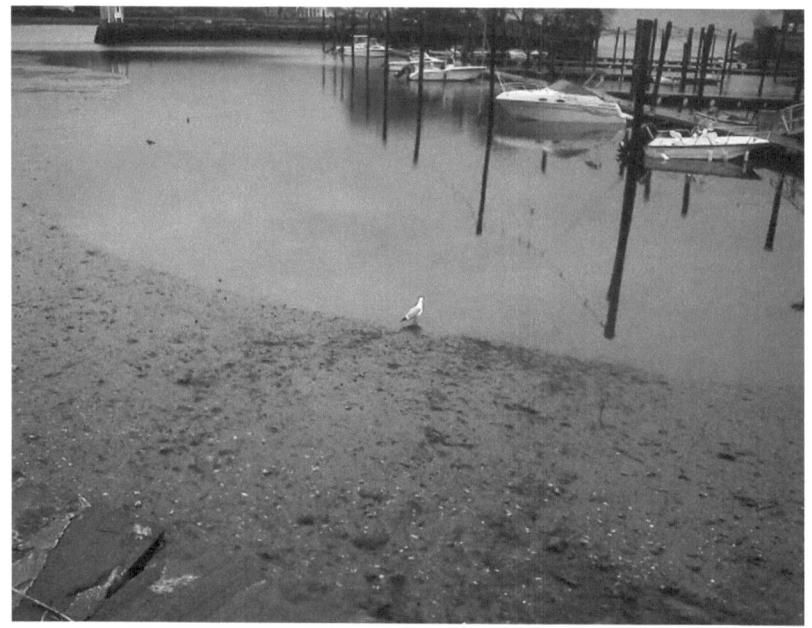

Next she heard a voice and it told her, "Belle, please pay attention to the number

4"

After being startled, Belle thought of the four seasons, the four directions and then she thought about four special things that the Native American kid and the Chinese kid and the kid from India all talked about in their own way –

The four special elements of nature

Earth

Air

Fire

Water

And just then Belle knew something special was going to happen.

She slept like a baby all night long.

She paid special attention to nature on her very special vacation.

The Earth

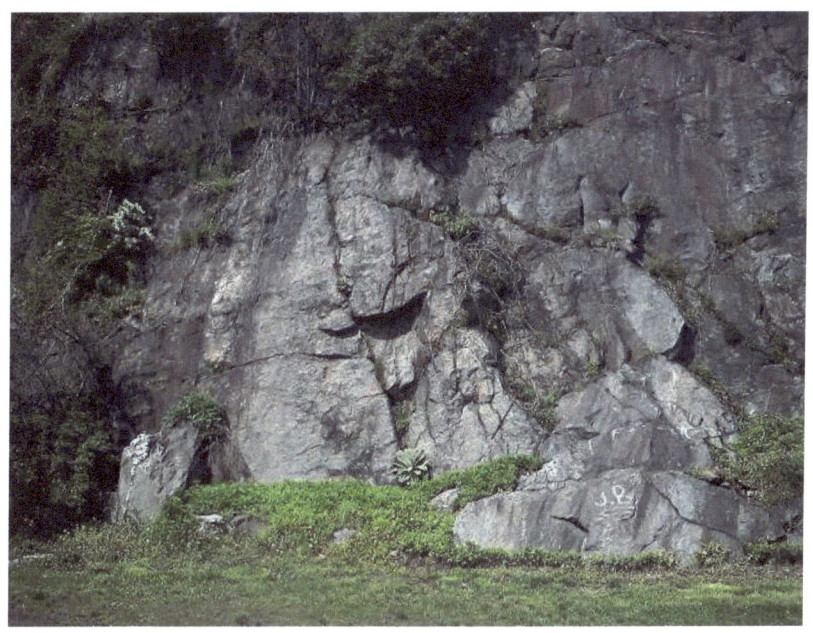

Even just looking at the earth can make us feel solid and strong. It's like we become that which we see – in a way we do! Check out the mirror neuron system to better understand why.

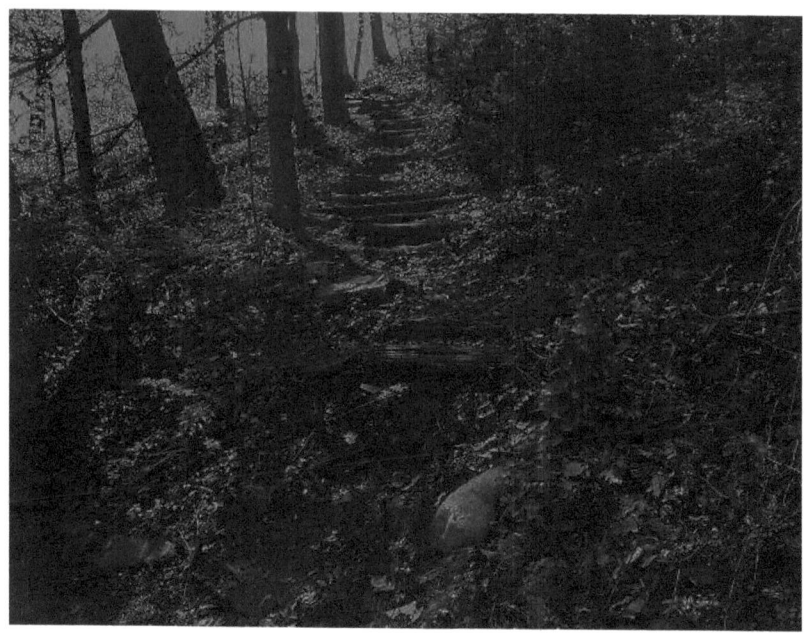

And when we might feel overwhelmed, and the goals unsurmountable, the Earth will sometimes show us a way - a shortcut to reach our goals from a different direction.

Sometimes we feel as though we are chained to the Earth. Scholars even think that past traumas and even past lives can keep us trapped to the Earth – you decide.

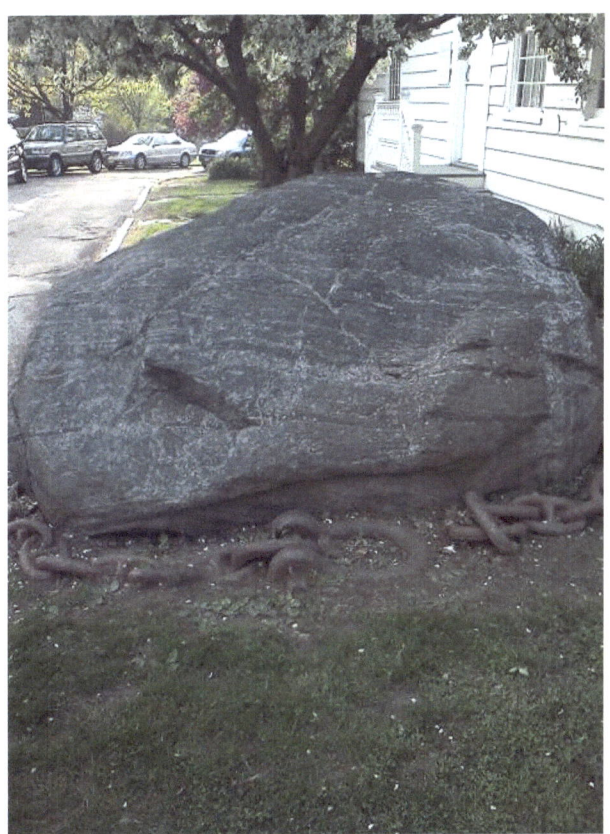

Our challenges may occur in pairs.

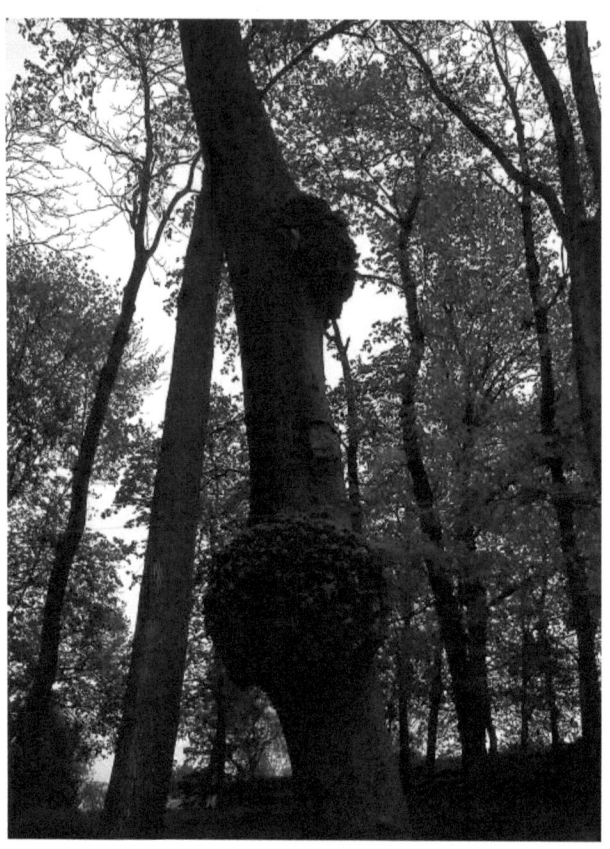

It is sometime a blessing to be given choices when the Earth provides us with new opportunities.

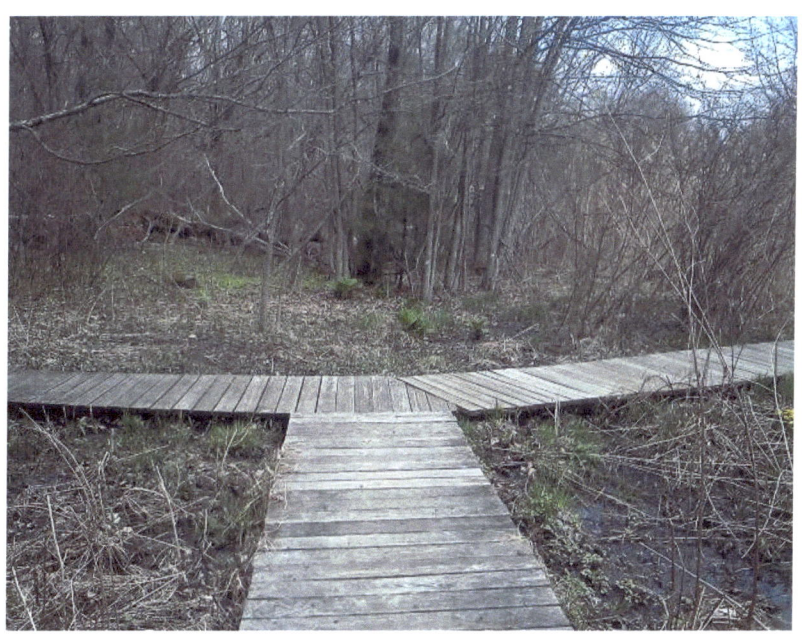

We may think we are trapped by the muck when all of a sudden a bridge appears giving us a new opportunity to pass over the problem.

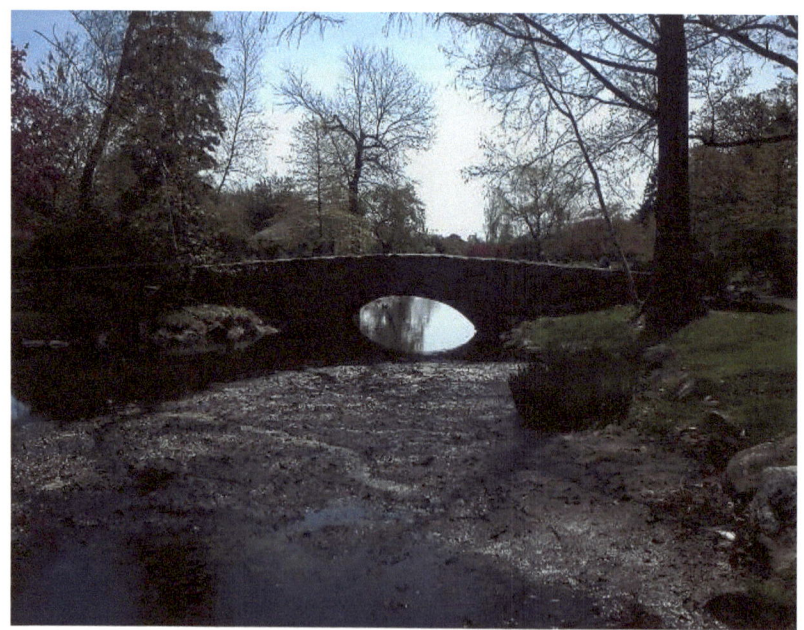

~ 14 ~

And new ideas are born.

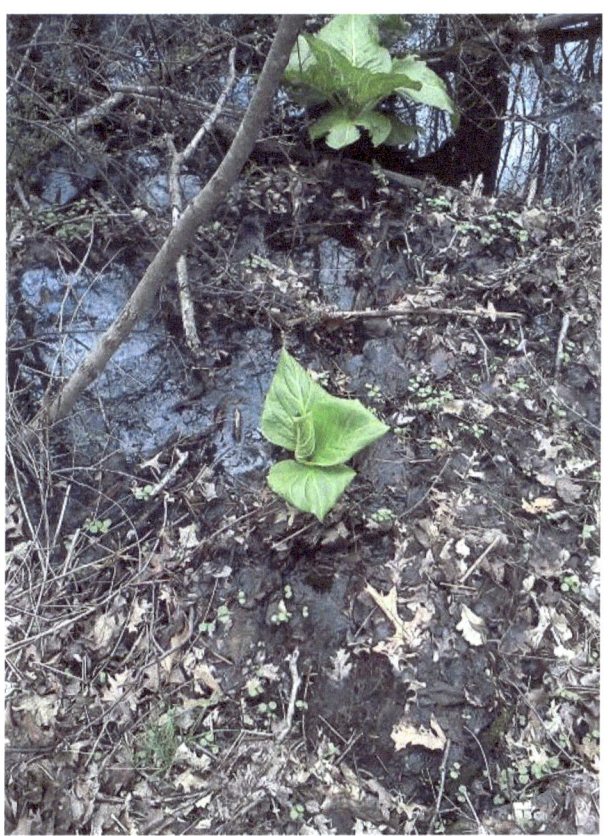

Air

Sometimes we need to look up and pay attention before we can better understand the direction we are traveling in.

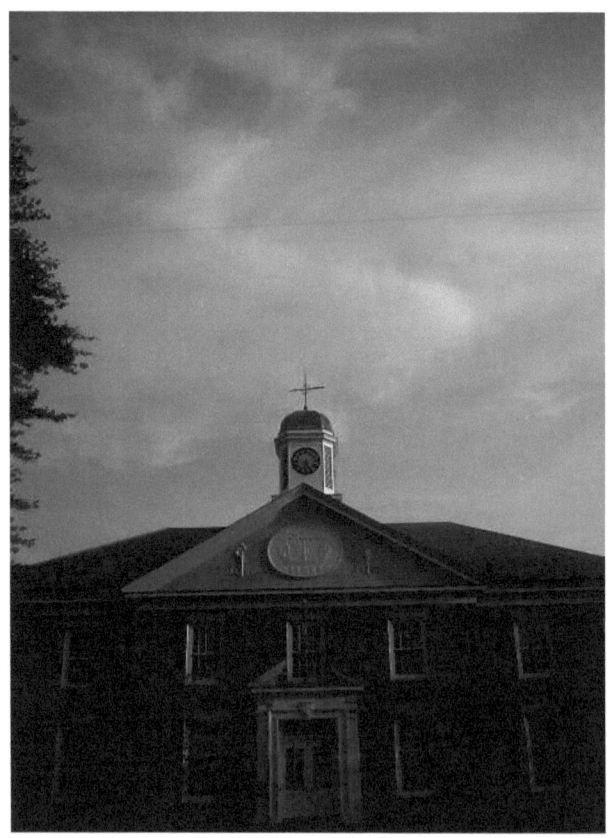

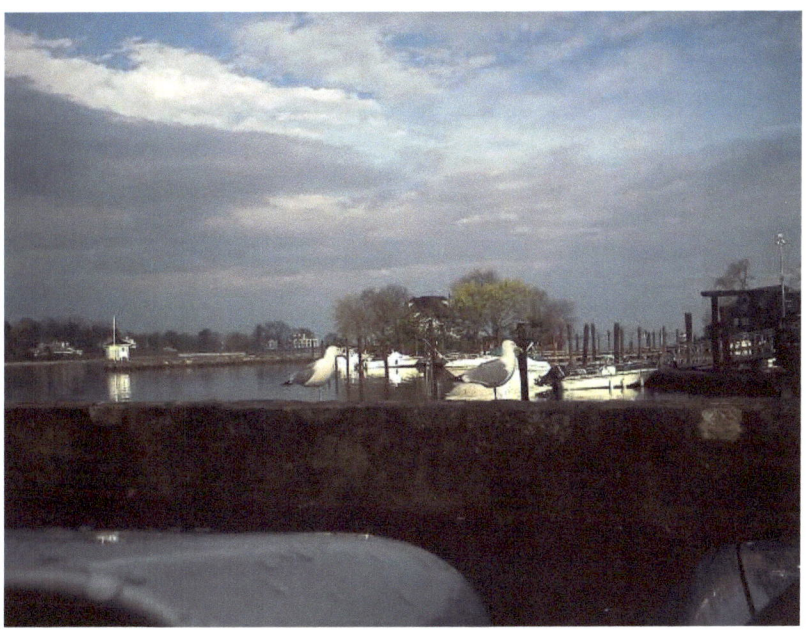

The clouds have a special connection with us. They just are and we just are as well. As we observe them moving and changing forms we can be detached and they can teach us how to relax by staying disconnected.

On the other hand, when we get too airy, we can forget about or miss important details that

~ 17 ~

are right in front of us – like the seagull in the picture above.

There is something real special about reaching and even living towards the sky. It builds confidence and security as we reach higher and higher.

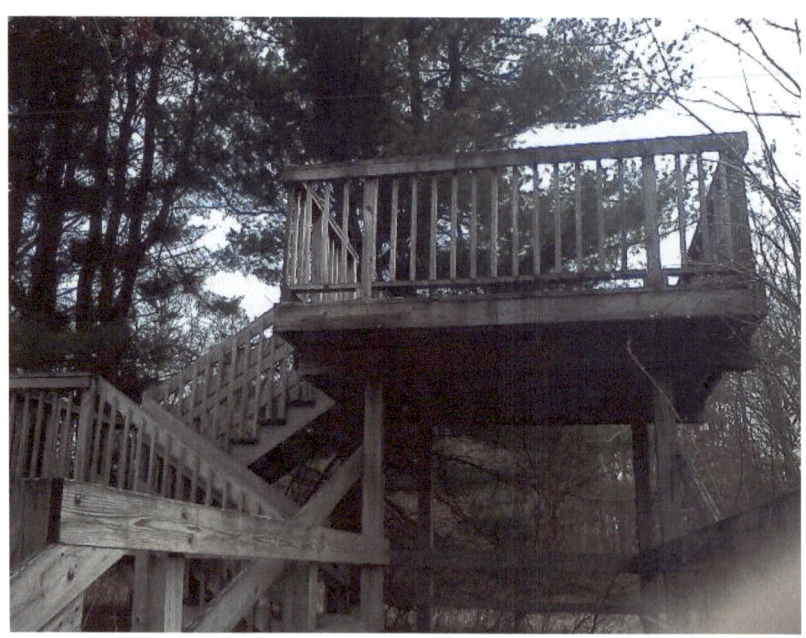

Fire

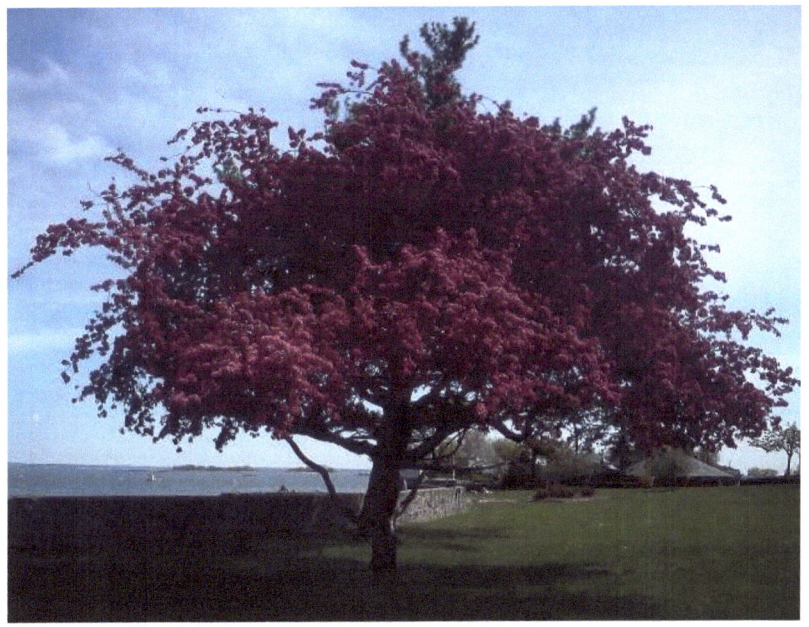

Color is very powerful - The color of fire and the fire of life gives us energy and motivates us to do things.

Sitting around a campfire can make us feel warm and safe and even more confident.

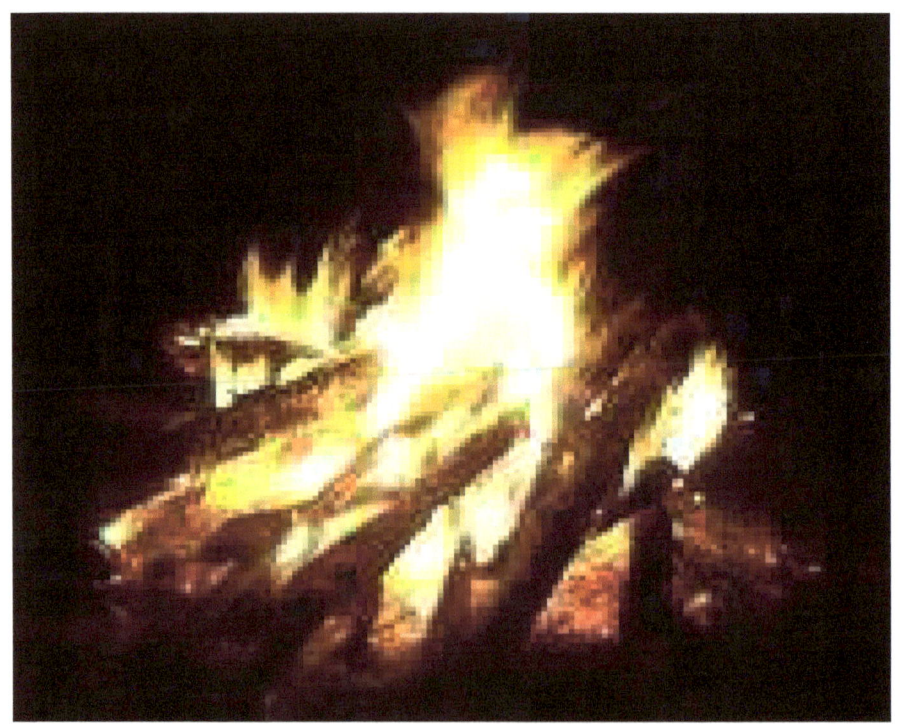

Some people even meditate on the somewhat steady colors and sounds within a campfire or a fireplace – it can make them relax and also make them invigorated.

~ 20 ~

And we learn to harness energy from the sun in many ways – new and not so new.

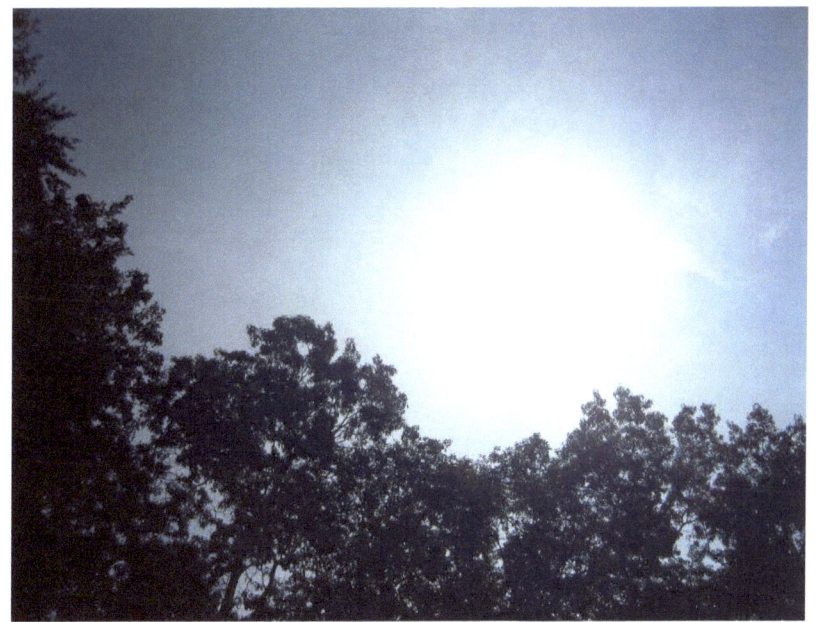

In new ways that are still from our nature - regardless of how we pretend otherwise.

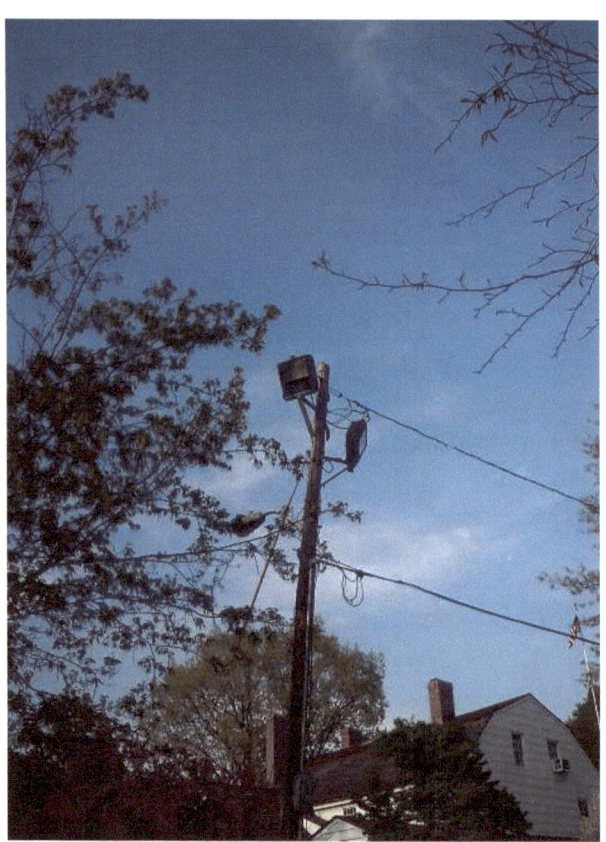

Water

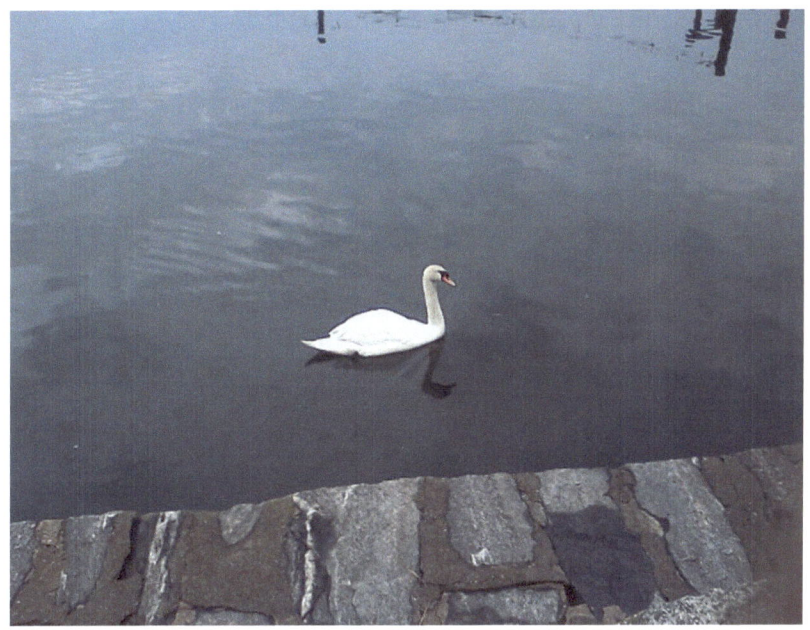

Water can be serene and soothing when we are under pressure – and don't worry so much about what's under the surface.

Even the sound of water can help us to when we are tired – they say that it even changes our brainwaves – how fast we process things.

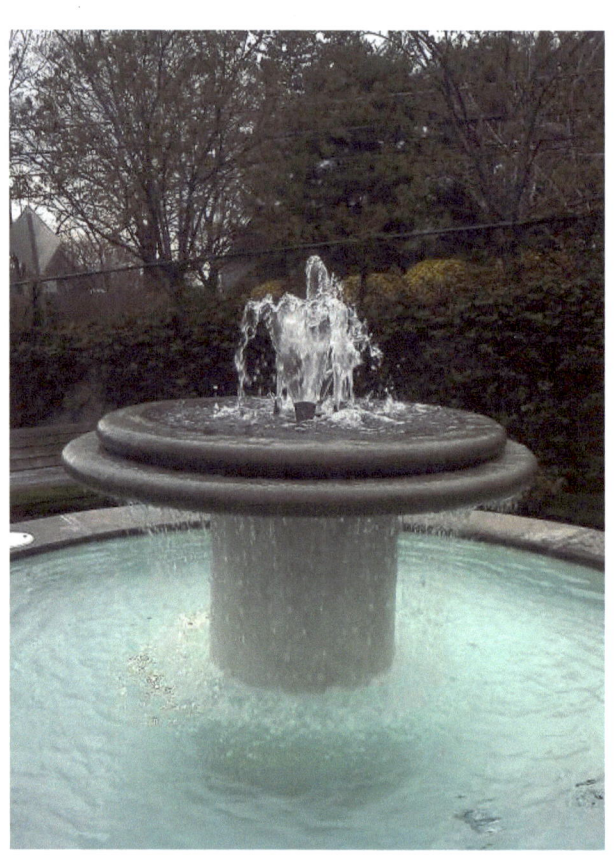

Swimming in sea water can make us strong and confident as the minerals are absorbed into our bodies and we make our muscles stronger.

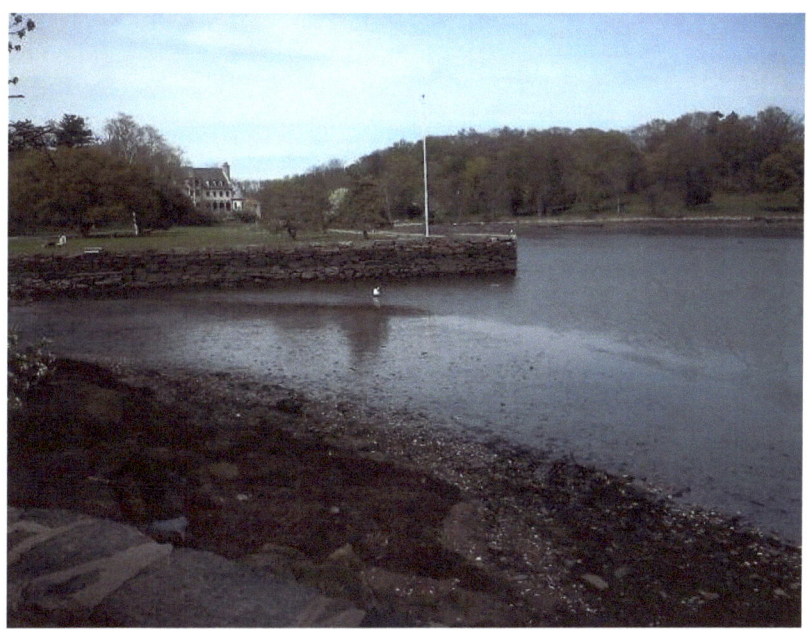

Water can provide a special type of healing for all creatures – even the most beautiful ones.

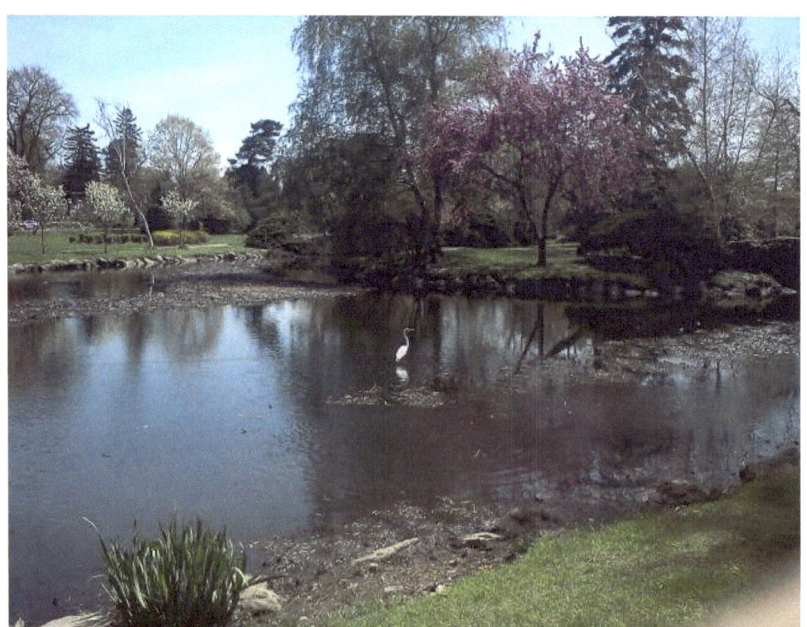

And Belle lived happily ever after as a child of the Earth, the Air, Fire and Water – but somehow she knew that she was something much grander than all of those things too.

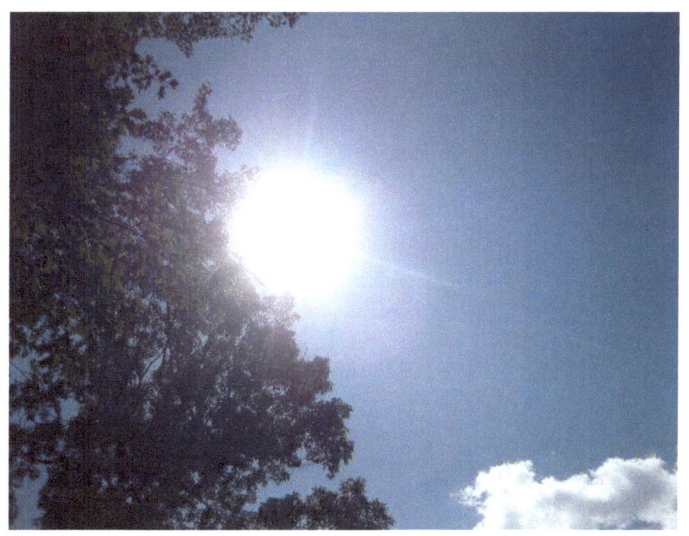

She was also a child of Spirit beyond the sun. She even slept better from that night on and had the most interesting of dreams from that day forward.

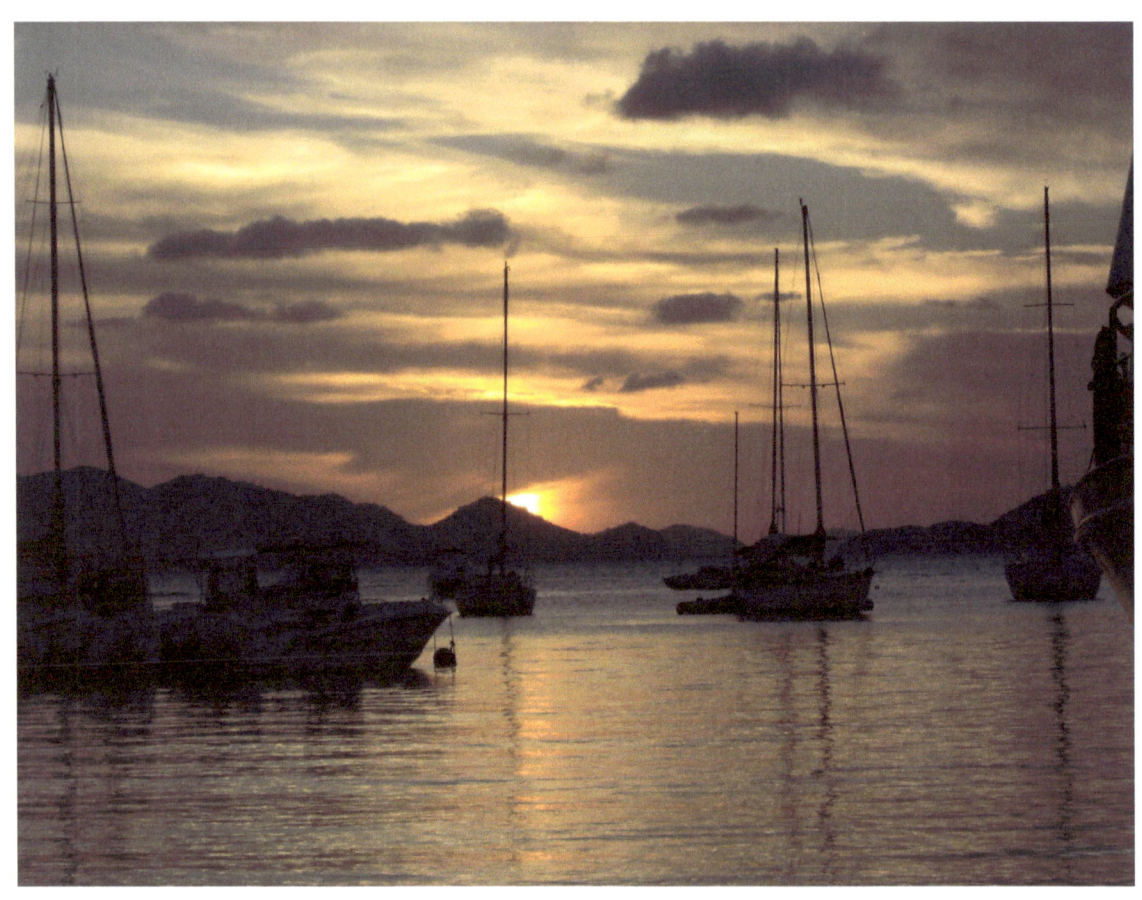

The Beginning

~

~ 28 ~

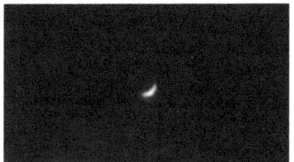

Workbook Section

It's OK to get help with this section

Please think of some ways that things from the Earth have helped you.

1)

2)

3)

4)

5)

Please write down some ways that you have benefited from the Air Element.

1)

2)

3)

4)

5)

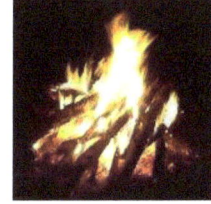What about the Fire Element?

1)

2)

3)

4)

5)

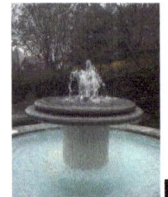How has the Water element helped you?

1)

2)

3)

4)

5)

Please think of some new ways that your family can be healed by cooperating with nature.

1)

2)

3)

4)

5)

Please think of some new activities related to nature that your school might benefit by.

1)

2)

3)

4)

5)

What are some new ways that we might harness clean energy from the sun, the air, fire or water?

1)

2)

3)

4)

5)

Notes

Notes

www.ingramcontent.com/pod-product-compliance
Lightning Source LLC
Chambersburg PA
CBHW041526280526
45792CB00004B/1393